Diabetes Diet: How to Eat Right to Beat Diabetes

The Complete Nutrition Guide for the Diabetes Diet

By: Raleigh Turner

9781632874528

I0413954

PUBLISHER'S NOTES

Disclaimer – Speedy Publishing, LLC

This publication is intended to provide helpful and informative material. It is not intended to diagnose, treat, cure, or prevent any health problem or condition, nor is intended to replace the advice of a physician. No action should be taken solely on the contents of this book. Always consult your physician or qualified healthcare professional on any matters regarding your health and before adopting any suggestions in this book or drawing inferences from it.

The author and publisher specifically disclaim all responsibility for any liability, loss or risk, personal or otherwise, which is incurred as a consequence, directly or indirectly, from the use or application of any contents of this book.

Any and all product names referenced within this book are the trademarks of their respective owners. None of these owners have sponsored, authorized, endorsed, or approved this book.

Always read all information provided by the manufacturers' product labels before using their products. The author and publisher are not responsible for claims made by manufacturers.

This book was originally printed before 2014. This is an adapted reprint by Speedy Publishing LLC with newly updated content designed to help readers with much more accurate and timely information and data.

Speedy Publishing, LLC©2014

40 E. Main Street #1156

Newark, Delaware

19711

Contact Us: 1-888-248-4521

Website: http://www.speedypublishing.com

REPRINTED Paperback Edition: ISBN: 9781632874528

Manufactured in the United States of America

DEDICATION

This book is dedicated to persons like me who struggle with diabetes on a daily basis. It can be a rough battle and it is a struggle to eat right and take the medications on time.

TABLE OF CONTENTS

Publisher's Notes   2

Dedication   3

Table of Contents   4

Introduction   5

Chapter 1- What Is Diabetes?   12

Chapter 2- The Effects of Malnutrition   15

Chapter 3- What Causes Diabetes?   19

Chapter 4- The Need for Supplements   24

Chapter 5- Herbs & Essential Fatty Acids   37

Chapter 6- A Look At Super foods   41

About The Author   49

INTRODUCTION

"All you need is a proper diet of fresh fruits and vegetables and get plenty of exercise and you'll be fine."

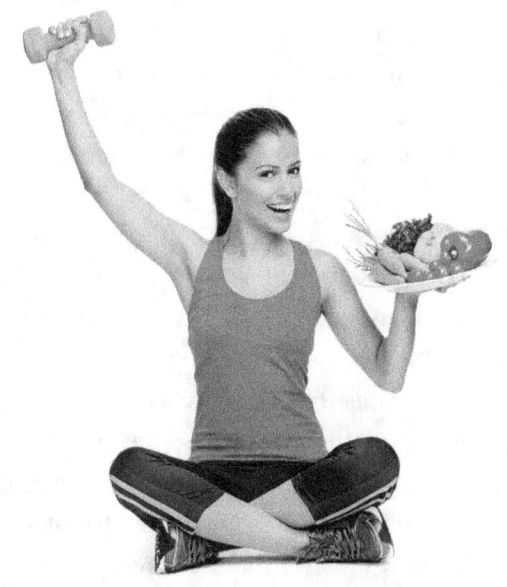

Ever heard those words from your doctor?

If that's all he/she recommends then you're missing out an important ingredient for health that he's not telling you. The fact is that you can adhere to the strictest diet, watch everything you eat and get the exercise of a marathon runner and still come down with diabetic complications. Diet, exercise and standard drug treatments simply aren't enough to help keep your diabetes under control.

Diet and exercise are the two words given out by established medicine and the media as the only cure-all; repeated endlessly like a holy mantra.

The word "fresh" is glossed over and likely you miss that word too. The simple truth is that what you buy from your supermarket shelves and bring home is not fresh. Those veggies look good on the outside, but they lack essential nutrient that everyone needs to maintain a healthy lifestyle, most especially those with diabetes. Without those nutrients, you are a prime target for degenerative diseases like Alzheimer's, cancer, heart disease and arthritis.

Those veggies on your store shelves come from farms whose soil has been depleted of vitamins, minerals and the antioxidants your body needs to maintain health. Today you'd have to chow down 17 bowls of spinach to get the same amount of nutrition that one bowl would have supplied 100 years ago. And along with this severe depletion come the herbicides, pesticides, additives and other treatments to those fruits and vegetables fresh and looking good before they get to your kitchen table. If that wasn't enough most of us live a hectic lifestyle that does nothing to help maintain good health. We smoke; we drink and eat far too much. Lack of exercise and sleep leads to high stress and depression. With all these factors combined and you have a recipe for disease and death!

While we live in fancy homes and drive the latest model car, we aren't happy. Our days are filled with doctor visits to repair the effects of a lifestyle we're often not willing or unable to change. Basically, a lifestyle change and not endless doctor visits is what we really need for proper health. And an understanding of how our bodies work is far more important than popping a Glyburide to control blood sugar. Medications alone will never cure diabetes. They are quick fixes and only treat the symptom.

But if you hope to survive the three most prevalent diseases of diabetes, heart diseases and cancer, the only cure is to address the things that you are doing that are making you ill. Certainly diet is an important ingredient. So is exercise.

While there is plenty of food to go around, the quality is poor. Eating organic food, referred to as "fresh" by your family doctor is essential. But many of us don't have a source where we can buy fresh food. And because you can't always eat fresh, supplementing is the only answer. This is the one word doctors leave out and you are ignorant of. Since there is no profit in suggesting you take chromium to control your blood sugar, your doctor leaves this essential information out. The result can be disastrous for you! Diabetic complications are a direct result of the lack of nutrients you can only find in fresh produce.

Many Americans today are not getting adequate amounts of vitamins and minerals in their diet. Many don't even meet the minimum RDA (Required Daily Allowance) as set by government health agencies. Likely you're one of those many. Your body needs vitamins and minerals to fight viruses, disease, bacteria and pathogens that invade you on a daily basis. If fresh fruits and vegetables were easy to acquire you wouldn't need the power of supplements.

That's where this book comes in. Whether you are currently in good health or are suffering from diabetes, supplementation is necessary! And as a diabetic, supplementing is an absolute necessity! Diabetics lose a great amount of nutrients that are flushed away in the urine. The kidneys are stressed as they try to rid your body of excess glucose. Unfortunately, a lot of vitamins and minerals get flushed down the toilet along with the glucose.

Your doctor likely hasn't told you about the importance of supplementation simply because he either doesn't know or has never learned about the importance of supplements or, if he does, he finds no profit in telling you. After all, drugs are what he prescribes and what puts money into his pockets. He knows next to nothing about prevention, nor does he know anything about natural alternatives to any health problems.

Unfortunately, this lack of education can lead you down the road to diabetic complications. And an early date with the coroner. Without essential nutrients, your body simply breaks down. It ages rapidly. Free radicals ravage the cells in your body, produce glycation and make room for diseased cells to proliferate.

Scurvy, for example, is the result of a lack of vitamin C. Diabetics lack adequate amounts of this vitamin. Chromium and vanadium are two other vital minerals lacking in diabetics. In fact, the lack of some essential vitamins and minerals it has been shown, lead to the following complications:

- Neuropathy. Diabetics often lose feeling in their hands and feet. The nerves die, not necessarily because of excess sugar in the diet, but because of a lack of vitamins and minerals which can help fight those complications. With deadened nerves there is no pain when stepping on a sharp object. Infection sets in and the wound festers. In all cases the wound does not heal or heals very slowly. If not treated, foot ulcers and gangrene set in. For many diabetics, amputation of the limb is the only solution. No amount of oral medication by your doctor can treat this problem. Even if you insure there are no sharp or rusty objects about, the lack of nerves makes it difficult to walk. Pain and tingling sensations are the signals that your nerves are about to die. Though your doctor may not say so, there is something you can do to prevent this from happening to you.

- Retinopathy. As with the deadening of the nerves in the feet, the same thing happens to those delicate veins in the eyes that lead the diabetic toward a future of blindness. It is preventable if you know what supplements you should take to avoid getting blinded.

- Kidney Disease: The kidneys are under great pressure as they try to rid your body of excess glucose. The higher your glucose level and the longer it stays in your blood, the harder the kidneys have to work. With so much pressure, they malfunction and disease can set in. More than half of all patients on dialysis today are diabetic.

- Heart disease. Your heart is hardly immune to the effects of high blood sugar. An ingredient such as CoQ10, so necessary for the proper beating function of the heart is depleted in the diabetic. If you take a statin drug to control your cholesterol, your chance of a heart attack is even greater. Statins are known to rob the heart of CoQ10.

These are just some of the complications that strike the diabetic. Clearly supplementation is necessary. But where do you find the information about which supplements you should take if your doctor knows nothing about them? The information is out there, but with a busy lifestyle you don't have time to read the hundreds of books on treating your diabetes.

That's why this book was written. Here you'll find the kind of information you need to supplement with the right kind of vitamins and with the right. No guesswork. If you are diabetic, the information here will provide you with an outline to get you started on the road to recovery.

Through generations, we have grown to trust and put our complete faith in our doctors.

Unfortunately, that trust is unfounded today. Your doctor is under pressure to sell drugs. Behind him stands a pharmaceutical company that collects billions of dollars in annual sales. Their focus is not to help get you well. Their focus is pure profit. And while your doctor may be well meaning, his hands are often tied and has to push drugs as the only solution to the disease.

Today's doctor studies many years in a medical school owned and operated by a pharmaceutical giant. Naturally, he studies drugs and knows which drug to prescribe for what ailment. Natural treatments and supplements are not taught. While he may want to see you get well, his practice is based on treating the sick and if he doesn't have enough sick people to treat, he's out of work! The doctor who attempts to actually help his patients rather than prescribe standard medication is at risk of losing his practice!

Starting a supplementation program is the best thing you can do to protect yourself against complications and you should discuss this with your doctor. But if he plays down the importance of supplementation, you might want to seek the aid of a naturopath or a dietitian who knows more about vitamins and minerals and can help you set up a good program.

This book focuses on all the essential vitamins, minerals, herbs and more to help fight your disease. Diabetes can be reversed, though, as yet, there is no cure. But remember that supplementation is just one of many changes you need to make if you hope to live a long and fruitful life. But remember that supplementation alone is not enough. It must be combined with the right diet, exercise program and especially the willingness to change the many bad habits that have led you to become ill. Those habits are not easy to change and won't happen overnight.

CHAPTER 1- WHAT IS DIABETES?

Diabetes is a blood sugar disorder. Excess glucose in the bloodstream doesn't get into the cells and muscle tissue of the body where it acts as fuel to be burned as energy. Diabetics often find themselves sluggish and tired.

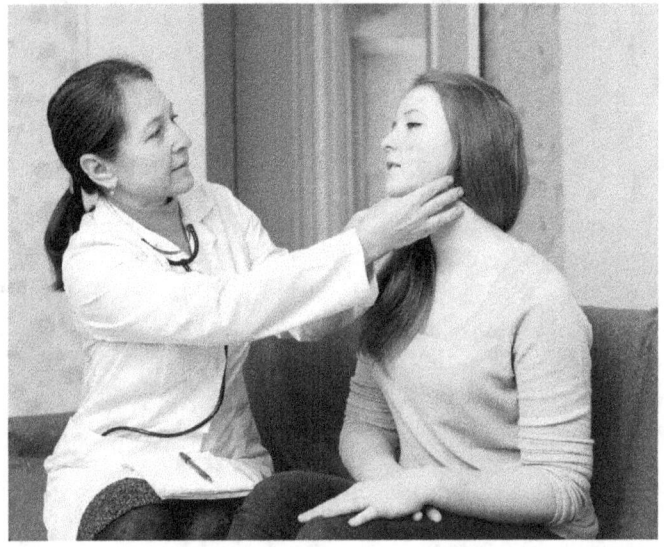

In order to get into the cells, glucose must have both insulin and GTF (Glucose Tolerance Factor). Insulin acts as a key. It opens the cell "door" so glucose can get in where it can be stored and used as energy. Insulin is generated by the beta cells of the pancreas. Under normal conditions the pancreas produces just enough insulin to get the job done. Insulin production occurs shortly after eating. Things are different for the diabetic.

The food you eat is turned into glucose. How much depends on the type of food and how much you eat. A meal high in simple carbohydrates will lead to a sharp rise in blood sugar. Complex carbohydrates take longer to be converted into glucose. The pancreas kicks in to produce insulin so the excess sugar can be shuttled into the muscle and other cells of the body for future storage and then be used as energy.

There are two types of diabetes. In type 1, the pancreas does not produce enough insulin to get that glucose into the cells. With little insulin to shuttle excess glucose into the cells, glucose stays in the bloodstream where it builds up to dangerous levels and begins to wreak havoc on the organs. Type 1 is usually prevalent in the early years and usually strikes children and young adults. The reason why the pancreas does not do the job of producing insulin is unclear, though it is assumed that the pancreas becomes damaged or is attacked by the body's own immune system. Cancer of the pancreas can contribute to a lack of insulin, though this condition is rare in children. Yet another reason is due to burnout which results to overproduction of insulin and eventual burnout of the pancreas.

Whatever the reason, Type 1 diabetics require insulin shots to do the job the pancreas cannot perform. They need to take insulin before every meal to control their blood sugar and require it for the rest of their lives. Only 5% of diabetics fall into the Type 1 category.

The majority of diabetics are Type 2. They have healthy pancreas that generates adequate amounts of insulin, but the insulin is not able to "open the door" of the cells so glucose can enter. To compensate, the pancreas produces more insulin to get the job done. But often the cells become resistant to insulin-they simply don't open up. This situation makes the pancreas produce even more insulin. Eventually, the pancreas cannot produce any more and burns itself out. Type 2 diabetics have no lack of insulin. The cells just don't recognize insulin.

Diabetes Diet

The reason for this insulin resistance is due to the fact that most type 2 diabetics are overweight and obese. Fully 90% of Type 2 diabetics are overweight or obese. It has been shown that fat around the abdominal region acts like a separate organ, producing compounds which can make cells resistant. Excess fat interferes with the functioning of the cells. Just by shedding a few pounds, you can better manage your blood sugar levels. Of course weight loss is not the only solution. Besides excess weight a sedentary lifestyle aggravates the problem. The cells need oxygen and the proper nutrients that make them elastic and better able to take in glucose. The proper amount of exercise helps them do the job.

The human body is made to be active. Without some kind of activity, whether it's as simple as walking, cooking or cleaning, cells can't function. A diet of highly refined and processed food loaded with fat and sugar makes up the standard fare of most everyone, but does little to help those cells.

Diabetes rates a close third behind heart disease and cancer. Many of the foods you buy come loaded with fat, sugar and salt and has little essential fiber like that of our early ancestors. It's the lack of the right nourishment that is leading the world to the epidemic of diabetes.

CHAPTER 2- THE EFFECTS OF MALNUTRITION

Our store shelves are stocked with an endless variety in taste, texture, sweetness and packaging.

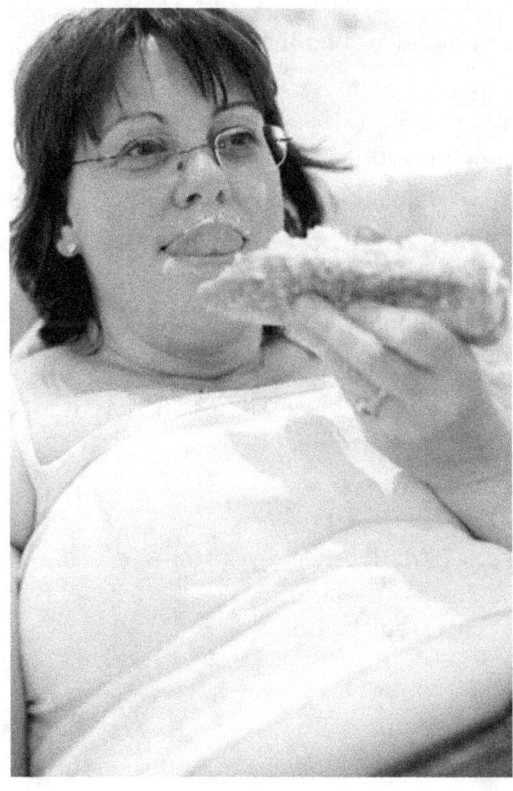

With so much food available it's hard to believe that many Americans are malnourished. While we sympathize with the poor in countries where food is scarce, we don't realize that famine can strike anywhere, even in the richest nations on Earth. We don't need to be undernourished to suffer from malnutrition, which is just another form of famine.

We grow enough food to feed ourselves and throw away enough food to feed 50 million people every day. There's enough food in storage to feed us all for a year if our nation's farmers decided to stop growing food.

Despite this food, wealth, we are seeing a rapid rise in degenerative diseases around the world.

As more nations adopt the Western-style diet, we see more diabetics where there once were few of them. All of this, it has been established, has been brought about by the poor choices of the food we eat. Taste, cost, convenience and gratification is the primary concern. But those choices do not provide the right kind of nourishment for health. White bread, coffee, beer, hot dogs and soft drinks are the primary food and drink consumed. Just take a look at this list of popular grocery items purchased today:

- Coke Classic

- Cigarettes; Marlboro and Winston

- Kraft processed cheese

- Pepsi

- Diet Coke

- Campbell Soup

- Budweiser beer

- Tide Detergent

- Folger's Coffee

- White bread

Nowhere on this list do you find fruits, vegetables or whole grain cereal. A study done by the U.S. Department of Agriculture of over 11,000 Americans showed that:

- 41% ate no fruit

- 82% ate no cruciferous vegetables (broccoli, spinach and the like)

- 72% ate no vitamin C rich fruits and vegetables

- 80% ate no vitamin A rich fruits and vegetables

- 84% ate no high fiber grain food.

Not an impressive list of food items. If the trend continues, America will destroy itself before any enemy could choose to invade it. America spends some 1.5 trillion dollars in medical care, more than any other nation and yet ranks among the highest in sickness and disease! Americans are woefully low in Vitamins A, C, D, E, K, B-6, riboflavin, folate and lack the essential minerals of calcium, potassium, magnesium, zinc, iron, chromium and selenium. Fiber from plant proteins, special fatty acids and complex carbohydrates are lacking in our diet. Fat, sugar, alcohol, caffeine, cholesterol, food additives and toxins from the environment combine to the health woes we see around us today. With so many poor choices, it's not surprising that we are faced with so many diseases, all of which could easily be prevented.

If we suddenly keeled over into a diabetic coma after the first sugar spike, most of us would scramble to make changes in our habits.

Diabetes Diet

Unfortunately it takes years of an unhealthy lifestyle before symptoms start to show up. The first cigarette won't kill you, neither will that first hamburger. But constant habits are what translate into heart disease and diabetes.

While we live in expensive homes, drive the latest model car and own the latest electronic gadgets, disease of any kind won't allow us to enjoy it all. Clearly a lifestyle change is necessary, but few people have the self-discipline to make those changes.

CHAPTER 3- WHAT CAUSES DIABETES?

While diabetes is a blood sugar disorder, there are many factors that can lead to a diagnosis of diabetes. Some of them are:

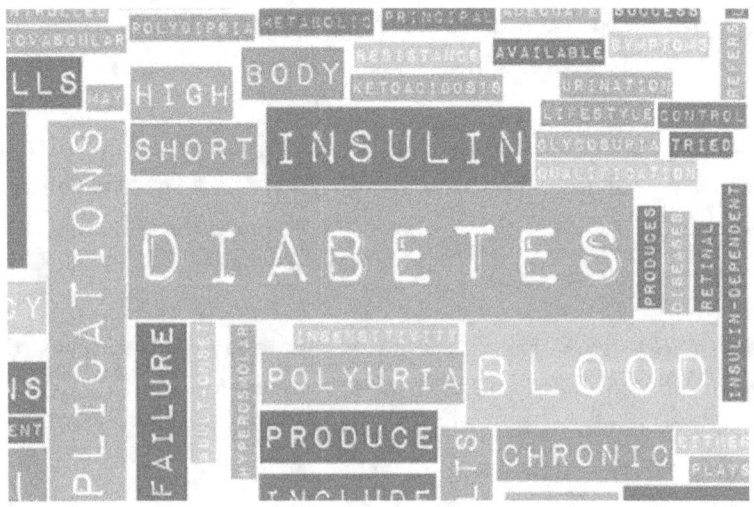

The Psychological Aspect: Many diabetics experience depression and a feeling of hopelessness. A diagnosis of diabetes is akin to a sentence of death and can lead to depression. Grief and sorrow over the loss of a loved one has an effect on blood sugar. Constant grief can lead to diabetes. The mind is a powerful mechanism and far from being separate from the body, it helps maintain health and can help to prevent disease or stem the onset of many diseases.

It's been shown that happy people get sick less. When you are happy, your brain secretes endorphins, the happy hormones. Being happy has been shown to improve the functioning of the body and regulate blood glucose level. How you view your world can determine the state of your future health. You can take all the vitamins, minerals and herbs to help your condition, but if you are bitter, angry and resentful, little of it will help.

Our Toxic Environment: We live among toxins of every kind. Whether it's in the air we breathe, in our fluoridated water supply, or the pesticides in our food, our bodies build up toxins which are hard to remove. Prescription drugs are made up of chemicals and add to the toxic burden. Alcohol and tobacco add fuel to the fire. This makes us weaker and less able to cope with the disease.

Malnutrition: Our bodies need certain nutrients in order to function properly. Since most of us are not getting enough essential nutrients in our diets, we are leaving ourselves vulnerable to diseases which otherwise could be overcome.

Lack of Exercise: Exercise aerates the body and supplies the organs, tissue and blood with needed oxygen. Our cells become more resilient and are better able to accept glucose with the help of oxygen. We are meant to be active. Most of us breathe shallow and take few deep breaths. A decent exercise program should be 30 minutes of any activity. Aerobics, walking, swimming, gardening can get the heart pumping. It's one of the best ways to stay healthy. As you get older, you tend to exercise less.

Age onset diabetes strikes many over the age of 40.

Diet: The food we eat is killing us. We consume what is fast and convenient, food that lacks the essential nutrients and fiber we need to motor through an active day. Processed food lacks fiber and leads to blood sugar spikes after meals, creates insulin resistance and makes us fat. Our highly refined food contains more fat, sugar, salt and additives and doesn't fill us up, so we eat more.

Supplements: It's forgotten in medical circles. Until the world can find a way to grow fresh produce and get it to your dinner table, supplements are a necessity. The lack of nutrition in our food supply demands supplementation. We cannot function properly without adequate amounts of vitamins and essential minerals to help fight disease and stay healthy.

Immune Function: There's no question that our current lifestyle is compromising our health. In order to have a functioning immune system to tackle the variety of viruses and bacteria out there, we need top performance. Today you don't need to be HIV positive to compromise your immune system. Most of us have already compromised our immune systems, making it easy for viruses to take hold. Smoking, excessive use of drugs and antibiotics makes it easy to get sick. May viruses mutate and adapt to our medical onslaught so new super strains take hold. The next virus to come along to kill us won't be any new unheard of disease, but one we could easily have overcome had we let our immune system do what it does best, instead of interfering with its functioning. There are some 20 trillion immune cells in your body that are helping to kill bacteria, viruses, yeast and cancer cells. We have the arsenal to help maintain health, we don't have the patience to let the inner workings of the body do its job.

Organ deficiency: There's little you can do with an existing heart defect that's due to hereditary factors. As we age, our organs become less efficient. Free radicals have a better chance to do damage.

One way to help is through the use of vitamins, minerals and herbal supplements. As you get older, you'll need supplements to help you fight the damage. Diabetics age faster than others simply because adequate amounts of basic nutrients are absent.

Chronic Infection: Infection in healthy individuals last a short while and disappear. Chronic infection is a sign that your body does not have the ability to rid itself completely of the infection. By pumping medications, you only mask, but don't get rid of the infection. So it returns again and again, better able to cope with the treatments you give it. The number one reason why people see their doctor is over the common cold. Sniffles and sneezes are something no one likes, but it is a sign that our bodies are purging something from our system. Rather than let our bodies handle it the way it was designed, we take a plethora of antihistamines, aspirins and drugs that do little to eliminate the virus. A chronic condition weakens your body and can lead to a diagnosis of diabetes.

Aging: No one gets any younger. By age 65 the average American has consumed 50 tons of food. With so many years of consuming highly processed food laced with chemical preservatives, aging occurs faster, and with it comes the diseases of aging. Osteoporosis, Arthritis, Alzheimer's, Parkinson's and cancer become the hallmarks of age. But the fact is, none of that has to happen. In some parts of the world, people live for a hundred years and maintain their energy and zest. Disease is not inevitable as the media would have you believe. The risk of developing diabetes doubles over the age of 40. We could live much healthier lives will into old age if we chose to take the necessary steps.

Oxygenation: Your body needs oxygen. A life in the big city breathing car exhaust and industrial pollutants only helps to starve our bodies and render it incapable of fighting disease. Our breathing is shallow. We breathe from the lungs. Proper breathing comes from the abdomen. You'll know if you are if your chest, rather than your abdomen, rises after you take a breath. Our red blood cells need oxygen and are heavily dependent on iron, copper, B-6, folate, B-12, proteins and zinc which cannot easily be

Raleigh Turner

assimilated without oxygen. Smoking robs you of the oxygen your body requires.

The fact is that without oxygen, no one can survive more than a few minutes. Obviously, lack of the proper amounts of oxygen is going to shorten your life. Cofactors like CoQ-10 and B vitamins improve the aerobic energy in cell mitochondria and oxygen plays a great part in getting it there. The good fatty acids in our diet help maintain the fluidity of cell membranes, which are better able to absorb oxygen and glucose.

Injury: Injuries take a long time to heal if your health is compromised. A long standing injury can lead to chronic infections and disease. New cell growth is blunted when there is not enough nutrients to help in the repair of the injury. If it takes too long for an injury to heal you are susceptible for diabetes after the injury takes too long to heal.

CHAPTER 4- THE NEED FOR SUPPLEMENTS

America and many parts of the world are deficient in many of the essential nutrients for vibrant health. Heart disease, cancer, diabetes and many other degenerative diseases are taking a toll on the health of millions around the world as they subscribe to the American diet. As the months and years pass, more strains and new diseases surface; old diseases such as tuberculosis are making a comeback. So many ill people cost billions of dollars in lost wages, sick time and production. Medical costs are skyrocketing.

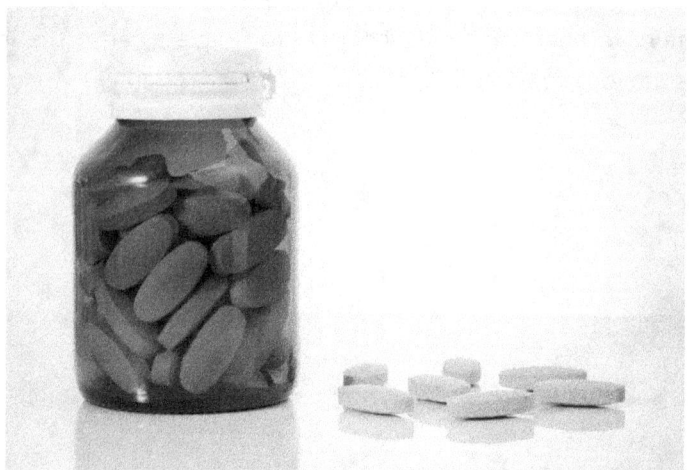

With the lack of nutrients in our food grown from commercial farms where the soil has been depleted and the herbicides and pesticides and other treatments used to keep produce fresh and looking good, everyone needs to supplement.

Here you'll find the essential supplements as are needed for the diabetic, from vitamins, minerals to valuable herbs and other foods to help you maintain health. Don't be easily swayed by media hype that certain vitamins and minerals are unimportant or are projected as being harmful. Most "studies" that claim that some nutrients are ineffective or dangerous are often flawed. Most "studies" are funded by big pharmaceutical companies that would rather see you use drugs as the only solution to handling your disease. For example, some studies pose that vitamin-E does little good. What the studies don't point out is that the synthetic form of the vitamin doesn't help you. If all the reports that minerals are bad for you then you would expect the CEO's of the big pharmaceutical companies to survive on burgers, fries and shakes. And you know that's never going to happen! All vitamins and minerals are essential.

Vitamins

Vitamins have an essential part to play in the maintenance of health and in the healing process.

Man throughout history has survived with only the vitamins and minerals that were abundant in the foods they ate and they found them in nature's own pharmacy. Thousands of studies have proven the usefulness of all vitamins.

While most of us fall short of the RDA requirements for optimum health, diabetics are worse off. If you lack certain vitamins, you will suffer the same symptoms as a diabetic. It is estimated that there are some 2 billion people who can be classified as having "syndrome X". They exhibit some form of insulin resistance. While they are within normal blood sugar range, their pancreas is producing far more insulin than the average rate. In other words their pancreas is overproducing insulin in order to keep blood sugar stable. And the primary reason is due to a lack of essential nutrients.

Diabetes Diet

Vitamins are safe. 400,000 Americans die every year from tobacco use and another 125,000 die from the side effect of prescription drugs, but no one has died from ingesting too many vitamins.

Let's look at some of the most important vitamins crucial to the survival of the diabetic and the non-diabetic alike:

Vitamin C: Vitamin C is a molecule similar to glucose and like glucose it needs insulin to get into the cells. Even if they take adequate amounts of the vitamin, diabetics still exhibit a deficiency of vitamin C. If you are diabetic, you need to take much more of this vitamin than the average person. A lack of this vitamin leads to scurvy-like symptoms: Poor wound healing, less immunity to infections, excessive bleeding, elevations in cholesterol and a depressed immune system. Vitamin C is required for proper immune function and the manufacturing of collagen, the main protein substance of the body. Taking Vitamin-C helps maintain the elasticity and function of the blood vessels and helps maintain proper blood pressure control. It has a mild effect on improving blood sugar control. While supplementing is necessary, it should not be used as an excuse for not eating foods that are rich in this vitamin.

Supplements alone, though cannot replace the high fiber, low fat and other healthy nutrients found in fresh fruit and vegetables. A supplement of 2000 milligrams has been shown to reduce the glycosylation (the tanning) of proteins in the blood) and helps avoid the toxic accumulation of sorbitol inside the cells.

Evidence shows there is a correlation between overweight people and the lack of Vitamin-C. The lower the level of vitamin-C, the greater the chance that you will be overweight. Those who have adequate levels tend to burn off 30% more fat during exercise than someone with low levels of C. Since diabetics are largely overweight and need to shed pounds, low C levels work against them. C is high in anti-oxidants that help against the rapid aging that occurs due to free radical damage in the body. While citrus fruits contain a good amount of vitamin-C, vegetables such as broccoli, bell peppers, potatoes and Brussels sprouts are also excellent sources.

Apples are an excellent source of Vitamin-C, quercitin and pectin. One Finnish study showed that those who ate the most apples and other foods high in quercitin had a 20% less chance of dying from diabetes and heart disease. The old adage that "an apple a day keeps the doctor away" still holds true today.

Vitamin E: This important vitamin acts as an antioxidant to protect against the dangers of damage to cell membranes. Nerve cells are most vulnerable, particularly the delicate nerves found in the eyes and feet. Little to no sensations in the feet and blindness are two common symptoms of diabetes.

Vitamin E has also been shown to:

Prevent free radical damage from LDL (bad) cholesterol and the damage to vascular linings.

- Improve the function of blood vessels and the cell lining themselves.

- Increase magnesium concentration within the cells

- Decreases levels of C-reactive proteins and other inflammatory compounds.

- Increases levels of glutathione, important for the antioxidants within the cells

- Improve the rate of electrical impulses in the nervous system

- Improve blood flow to the eyes.

- Improve kidney function and normalizes creatine clearance.

Be sure to take the natural form of the vitamin. Natural vitamin-E has a "d-" designation as in alpha tocopherol. "Dl-" is the synthetic form. Your body only recognizes the natural form. The synthetic version has been shown to retard the absorption of the real vitamin-E.

B Vitamin Complex:

Niacin B-3: Niacin helps in the burning of calories and, like chromium, is an essential component of GTF (glucose tolerance factor) that helps move glucose through the cell membrane. It has been shown to lower the need for insulin in type 1 diabetics, sometimes reversing the early onset of the disease. It helps improve beta function in the pancreas and improves blood glucose regulation. The best form of niacin is inositol hexaniacinate which helps reduce fats in the blood and has been shown to reduce cholesterol levels by 18%, triglycerides by 26% and increase the good HDL cholesterol by 30% when 1800 to 3000mg is used daily. However, if you suffer from gout, liver disease, peptic ulcers or hepatitis you should consult your doctor before taking Niacin supplements. Niacin's effect is enhanced with Vitamin-C.

Niacinamide is another B-3 vitamin and while niacin helps in lowering your cholesterol levels, niacinamide is used primarily to treat osteoarthritis and rheumatoid arthritis. 150-200 mg should be taken before a meal 3 times daily.

Vitamin B-6: Known as pyridoxine it helps balance triglyceride levels and normalize cholesterol levels. B-6 plays a part in the chemical transmitters in the nervous system, red blood cells and prostaglandins. Supplementation with B-vitamins helps fight nerve damage which is common among diabetics. Most diabetics are deficient in B-6. It also is beneficial for gestational diabetes, brought on by pregnancy.

Vitamin B-12 and Folic Acid: One of its uses is to reduce the pain of headaches, arthritis and the pain from dental surgery. Deficiency of this vitamin leads to the onset of neuropathy and increase serum levels of homocysteine. Taking the drug metformin lowers your vitamin B-12 stores, so you should have your serum levels checked every 6 months while you are on the drug. Taking this important vitamin will reduce the chance of coronary heart disease. Studies have shown that taking Folic acid along with B-6 and B-12 help to reduce homocysteine levels and clean out artery plaque. You can lower your homocysteine levels by eating less meat and other methionine-rich food.

Quasi-Vitamins

Although not considered essential, they do have a place to play in your health. Supplementing with them will add more protection.

Lipoic Acid: As we age, we produce less of lipoic acid. But lipoic acid works as an antioxidant with the ability to penetrate both fat-soluble and water-soluble areas of the body. It helps prevent the binding of sugar molecules to certain proteins in the boy, cell membranes and nerve tissue. It improves blood flow to the extremities of the body, such as the hands and feet. It's cousin, alpha lipoic acid is a small molecule that is easily absorbed and crosses cell membranes. It can quench both water and fat soluble free radicals inside the cell and outside. It extends the biochemical life of vitamin C and E and other antioxidants. It's considered an approved drug in Germany for the treatment of neuropathy and has been used successfully for the past 30 years. The nerves in the eyes are also susceptible which often leads to blindness in the diabetic. ALA can:

- Neutralize free radicals, primarily responsible for the aging process

- It is quickly absorbed and used by the body cells

- It is concentrated both inside and outside of the cell membranes

- Promotes normal gene expression

- Chelates metal ions and helps to eliminate toxic minerals from the body.

Quercetin: Citrus, berries, onions, parsley, legumes and green tea are loaded with bioflavonoids, which are used by the plants to help in the photosynthesis process and protect them against the damaging rays of the sun. There are some 500 varieties with some 20,000 estimated bioflavonoids. Quercetin is just one of them.

The best sources of quercitin can be found in the rind of citrus fruits, onions and apples.

Quercitin helps:

- Inhibit inflammation

- Is a potent oxidant

- Inhibits the fragile nature of capillaries that protects connective tissues against breakdown.

Raleigh Turner
- Reduces the stickiness of cells

Grape Seed Extract: Bioflavonoids are made up of some 20,000 chemical compounds and may be more important than vitamin C and ALA. Grape seed extract is a natural antihistamine. Its flavonoids inhibit allergic reactions that can cause eczema. It's a potent chelator that helps the body to remove toxins from the body. The dosage is at 100 mg 3 times daily. It contains:

- Anthocyanins which give black grapes, beets, red onions and berries their color.

- Catechins, also found in apples.

- Ellagic acid, an anti-cancer compound found in raspberries, cranberries and other berries

- Flavones, found in citrus fruit, red grapes and green beans

- Flavonols, such as quercitin, myricetin, found in spinach, kale, onions, apples and black tea

- Flavanones such as hesperidin found in grapefruit, oranges and lemons

Grape seed extract is closely related to pycnogenol, derived from the bark of pine trees. Pycnogenol helps to keep collagen elastic and softens the blood platelets so they move more efficiently.

Recommended dosage for pycnogenol is 400 mg.

L-Carnitine: There is no carnitine found in plant food, but red meat contains the most content. L- carnitine is produced by the body, but a lack of vitamin C, iron, niacin and B-6 lead to a deficiency. Lack of L-carnitine leads to a buildup of fats in the blood, liver and muscles. Symptoms of weakness are the usual result. Taking L-Carnitine induces the burning of fat within the cell's energy makers, the mitochondria. It lures fat into the cells where it can be burned for energy. It also helps you recover quickly from fatigue. Combined with vitamin-E, it is effective in combating heart disease. Taking 500 mg twice a day on an empty stomach is recommended. Anyone who is sick and stressed should take it. Children, the elderly and diabetics all benefit.

CoQ10: With prolonged use, statin drugs steadily rob the heart of this essential nutrient. Your heart needs CoQ10 for its proper beating function. Years of statin drug use often lead to heart attacks. While the body produces its own CoQ10, supplementation is critical if you are taking a statin. It is a powerful antioxidant and has the ability to trigger beta-cell function in the pancreas that helps to produce more insulin leading to better sugar control. CoQ10 helps lessen heart damage and retards the aging process. 50 to 100 mg per day is necessary to prevent the depletion in the body tissues and heart muscle when taking a statin drug. It should be taken with food. Here are its benefits in summary form:

Provides oxygen to tissues to help them heal better

- Triggers beta-cell function in the pancreas

- Lessens heart damage

- Retards the aging process.

Minerals

Minerals are an essential part of every diet. And the diabetic needs particular minerals if he is to avoid the complications that always arise as a result of the lack of nutrients. Without minerals, our bodies could not function as efficiently. Sadly, many Americans are woefully deficient in several minerals and because of poor dietary habits. The diabetic is extremely vulnerable to blindness, fatigue, and poor circulation. The best cholesterol lowering minerals are chromium, calcium, magnesium, selenium and zinc.

Chromium: 90% of Americans do not get 50mcg (micrograms) of chromium a day. The Food and Nutrition Board of the National Academy of Sciences considers 50 to 200mcg to be necessary. As a diabetic you need at least 200 to 400mcg a day. Chromium works with insulin in helping open the cell membranes to accept glucose. Without it, insulin's action is blocked. Its GTF (glucose tolerance factor) is the crucial molecule that helps speed excess glucose into the cells. It not only improves insulin's action to get into the cells, but it has been shown to decrease fasting blood glucose levels, improve glucose tolerance and decrease cholesterol and triglyceride levels as well as the HDL, good cholesterol.

Cheese, legumes, beans, peas, whole grains and molasses are good sources of chromium. The best source is brewer's yeast. However the taste of brewer's yeast makes it hard to take, so sprinkling it with your breakfast cereal or mixed in orange juice is a better way to take it. Chromium comes in many forms; chromium picolinate, chromium GTF and chromium enriched yeast are all suitable in your diet. The soils from most farms have been depleted of this essential mineral. It is crucial for proper blood sugar control. As most Americans are deficient in this nutrient, it explains the high incidents of obesity and the high number of people with Syndrome X whose blood sugars are normal, but who have a higher-than-normal rate of insulin production. Chromium GTF or chromium picolinate make good supplements.

Magnesium: Low intake of magnesium is a major risk factor that leads to retinopathy and heart disease in the diabetic. The RDA recommendation for healthy men is 350 mg per day and 300 mg for women. Between 300 to 600mg ideal. Many people only get between 143 to266 mg far short of the RDA standard. Our highly refined diet, lack magnesium. Magnesium, like chromium is involved in glucose metabolism. Supplementation has been shown to improve insulin response, glucose tolerance and improve the fluidity of red blood cell membranes in diabetic patients. Most magnesium comes from seeds, nuts, legumes, tofu and green leafy vegetables. You should take the highly absorbed form of magnesium such as magnesium aspartate or magnesium citrate. Take at least 25 mg of Vitamin B-6 per day to go along as this vitamin is linked with magnesium content in body cells. Without B-6, magnesium doesn't get into the cells and is otherwise useless.

Potassium: It's the major mineral inside of all cell membranes and its electrical charge generates what is called "membrane potential". It's believed that the ratio of sodium (which exists on the outside of the cells) to potassium is off kilter and this is one of the reasons why insulin cannot open the cell doors to accept glucose.

High potassium diets have been shown to lower the risk of many degenerative diseases such as cancer and heart disease and help improve glucose tolerance. Plant foods such as fruits, vegetables and whole grains serve as the best sources of potassium.

While a high intake of salt promotes high blood pressure, potassium counteracts this by helping lower blood pressure. Potassium supplementation can lower the systolic and diastolic blood pressure an average of 12 to 16 points. If you want to avoid salt, you can substitute with potassium as a safer alternative. NuSalt or No-Salt both contain potassium chloride and make good salt substitutes.

Generally supplementation of potassium is safe unless you have kidney disease.

Methyl Sulfonyl Methane: After water and sodium; MSM is one of the significant components in the body. It helps to control inflammation and muscle spasms, enhance blood flow and normalize the immune system. It's a crucial mineral for detoxification. Its an organically bound form of sulfur and found in small amounts in fresh plant food, though it is lost in cooking, storage and processing. Garlic, beans, eggs, cabbage, broccoli, and red peppers are good sources of MSM. Some of the advantages of MSM are:

- Blood glucose regulation

- Regular bowel movement

- Immune regulation

- Membrane fluidity

Manganese: Low insulin production in animals is due to a lack of manganese. Whole grains, fruits and nuts grown in well fertilized soil are good sources of manganese. It functions in many enzyme systems including those involved in blood sugar control and thyroid hormone function. It functions in the antioxidant enzyme superoxide dismutase (SOD). Diabetics have only half the manganese of normal people. A good daily dose of manganese for diabetics is 3 to 5 mg.

Zinc: This important mineral has a lot to do with various functions of the body from sexual development to immune functioning and maintenance of nerve tissue. Good sources of zinc are shellfish, organ meats, fish, pumpkin seeds, ginger root, nuts and seeds. Zinc deficiency leads to a loss of appetite. 10 to 60 mg per day is considered a safe dose. Too much can lead to copper deficiency and depress HDL cholesterol. Zinc is a cofactor in more than 200 different enzymes. Low zinc levels lead to infection, poor wound healing, a deficiency is taste and smell and skin disorders. It is involved with the secretion, synthesis and utilization of insulin and has anti-viral effects. It protects against the destruction of beta cells that produce insulin in the pancreas. Diabetics should supplement with 30 mg of zinc per day. Zinc along with vitamin-C and B-6 helps to speed up healing after surgery.

Vanadium: It's missing in the average American diet. In the form of Vanadyl sulfate it helps to control rises in blood sugar in diabetics. Before insulin was developed, vanadium was used primarily to treat diabetes. Good sources of vanadium are mushrooms, shellfish, dill, parsley and black pepper.

Chapter 5- Herbs & Essential Fatty Acids

Herbs

Bitter Melon: As the name implies it's not something easy to take. It's a cucumber like plant that grows in Asia, South America and Africa. Its strength lies in its ability to lower blood sugar. Just 2 ounces of the juice were shown to improve glucose levels in 73% of type 2 diabetics.

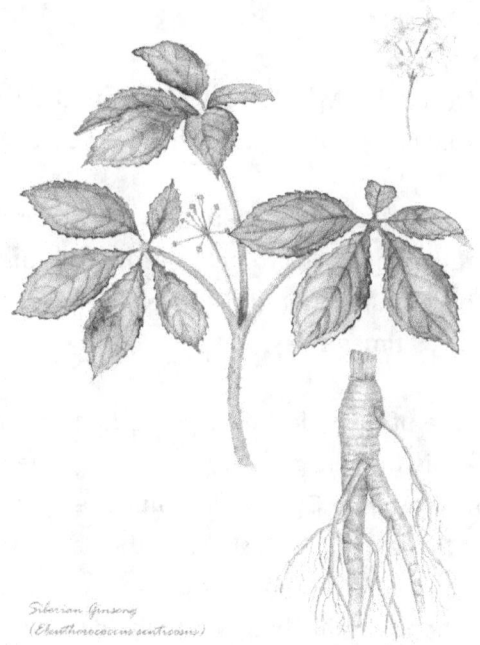

Siberian Ginseng
(Eleutherococcus senticosus)

Diabetes Diet

Gymnema Sylvestre: It's a plant that grows in tropical regions of India and was often used to treat both type 1 an 2 diabetics. In one study 400 mg of Gymnema extract was given to 22 type 2 diabetic patients along with their oral medications. All experienced improved blood glucose control and 5 of them were able to discontinue their drug use. Applied to the tongue, it has helped people eat fewer calories at a meal. It enhances the action of insulin. The dosage is 200 mg two times a day.

Fenugreek: The seeds were used in folk medicine to treat diabetes. In order to lower blood sugar, about 15 to 50 grams twice daily is needed. Considering the bitterness, it's not very palatable to swallow in capsules. A better use is as a condiment or spice like East Indians use. The active ingredient is the special soluble fiber of fenugreek along with the alkaloid trigonelline. It's helpful in both type 1 and type 2 diabetics.

Salt Bush: Native to the Middle East, 3 grams daily of salt bush provided improved blood sugar regulation in type 2 diabetes.

Bilberry: Known as European blueberry, it was used in France since 1945 to treat retinopathy. It protects the macula of the diabetic eye. Diabetics have found an improved version using supplements from 80 to 160 mg 3 times a day.

Ginkgo Biloba: One of the oldest living trees that has survived over 200 million years is the ginkgo. Very adaptable, one survived the nuclear blast in Hiroshima. Over a thousand scientific studies have been done over the last 40 years showing the value of ginkgo. The extract is widely prescribed in Europe today. It's an effective antioxidant. It improves the body's circulation and expands the small capillaries that nourish the extremities in the eyes, hands and feet. It inhibits the stickiness of cells, reduces inflammation and allergic responses.

Ginseng: One of the world's oldest herbs, it's considered an adaptogen that improves several body processes. Ginseng helps to lower blood pressure or raises it if it's too low. Just 3 grams before a meal can reduce after-meal blood sugar in type 2 diabetics. American ginseng helps by the stimulation of pancreas beta cells that leads to greater insulin output. Native Americans often used it. A type of Korean ginseng increases insulin sensitivity and helps lower blood sugar. One interesting side effect is an improvement in sexual function, something that many diabetics also suffer from.

Essential Fatty Acids

These are good fats that you find in fish, flaxseed, olive and canola oil, borage, evening primrose oil, lecithin, rice bran and rapeseed. Fish oil contains eicosaoentaenoic acid (EPA). EPA is prevalent in cold water fish like cod, salmon, mackerel, tuna and sardines. EPA has been shown to change the membrane fluidity of the body's cells, making it easy for them to accept glucose. It helps to prevent the stickiness of cells which can lead to heart disease and stroke. It also bolsters immune functioning and dilates blood vessels for better blood flow.

GLA: (Gamma linolenic acid): Borage, evening primrose and black currant oils are rich in this element. Corn fed beef contains a great amount of linoleic acid, which leads to tumor-producing acids. GLA helps as it is rich in prostaglandins that turn off the pain and stop inflammation. Native Americans dined on buffalo, which were free ranging animals and ate wild grains and seeds. The meat was lean and far healthier.

Diabetics lose the ability to make GLA in the body and as we get older we make less of it. Supplementation with 6 capsules of evening primrose oil, or one capsule of borage oil provide the 240mg needed for GLA requirements.

Diabetes Diet

CLA: Conjugated Linoleic acid is a collection of acids found mostly in the meat and milk of grazing animals. CLA is not found in plant food. A small dose of 3-4 grams have shown to help prevent breast cancer. Those who have cancer should take 1000 mg 6 times a day. The cooking process enhances CLA. So grilled beef has more CLA than raw. CLA has shown to:

- Improve glucose and insulin levels.

- Acts as an antioxidant.

- Suppresses arachidonic acid that causes inflammation

- Enhances the destruction of cancer cells and blocks the growth of tumors.

CHAPTER 6- A LOOK AT SUPER FOODS

While vegetables make up for essential eating, some foods come packed with a rich array of phytochemicals, vitamins, minerals, essential fatty acids and other nutrients that can help you in your battle to regulate your blood sugar. They're called Super foods because they contain rich levels of certain nutrients. Among them are:

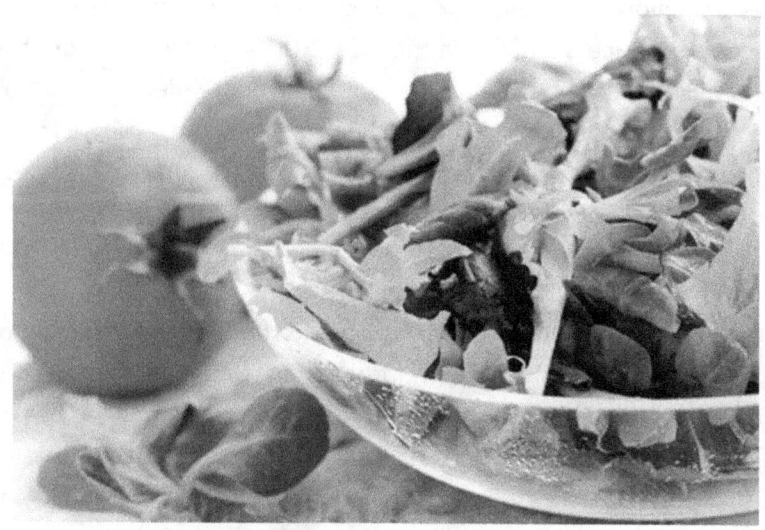

Fish and Flax Oil: Fish is one food that should be on everyone's plate at least once a week. It's rich in protein, B-6, B-12 and trace minerals and especially omega-3 fatty acids, severely lacking in the American diet. In one particular study those who consumed less than 1 ounce of fish daily had a significant reduction of glucose intolerance. Cold water fish such as salmon, halibut, sole, cod, tuna, trout and sardines can protect against the complications diabetes presents. Because they consist of protein, eating fish helps you feel full longer and fights the urge to snack. If you can't take fish every week, take a good fish oil supplement. Fish oil protects delicate cell membranes, which can better take in insulin and allow glucose into the cells.

Cold water fish has more omega 3 fatty acids. It was a staple in the diet of our ancestors. Our ancestors relied on a diet of a ratio of 1 to 1 in omega-3 to omega-6 fatty acids. Today, our ratio is unbalanced at 1 to 30 ratio of omega-3 to omega-6 fatty oils with extremely high levels of trans (hydrogenated) and saturated fats. With the saturated fats from margarine and beef, cell membranes become more rigid and can't recognize insulin and open up to receive the excess glucose in the blood. Unsaturated fats from fish and flax oil make those cell membranes more flexible. Flax oil contains alpha linolenic acid, which is converted into fish oil in the body. Both flax seed and flax oil contain good amounts of omega-3. You can bake with flax seed or sprinkle the seed into your morning cereal, or add it to ground beef for a leaner burger.

Garlic: Garlic, called the stinking rose is one of the miracles of nature. It has been used for centuries for its medicinal properties and healthful benefits. It belongs to the same family as leeks, onions, chives, scallions and shallots. Allicin is what gives garlic its distinctive odor. The oils enter the bloodstream and remain for several hours. Unfortunately, garlic breath is a nasty side effect, but chewing a sprig of parsley or a coffee bean helps eliminate the odor after eating. The source of the smell remains deep in the bloodstream where the garlic is producing its therapeutic effect and cannot be so easily be eliminated by using breath mints, toothpaste or mouthwash. Despite its odor, garlic should be on the plate of anyone who wants to stay healthy. It was eaten by the Israelite slaves who built the pyramids and garlic has been found in the tombs of Egyptian Pharaohs.

It's only in the past few decades that its healing qualities have been discovered. Whether aged, fresh, cooked or as a supplement it helps against liver damage, it modifies the extremes in blood sugar after a meal. You can buy odorless garlic supplements at your health food store. Odorless garlic products contain alliin and other sulfur compounds and provide all of the benefits of fresh garlic if they are manufactured properly. When looking for a supplement, look for an enteric-coated product as it does not break down as it passes through the stomach until it reaches the intestines. Stomach acids tend to destroy the alliin in garlic. Recommended brands of garlic are: Garlicin (Nature's Way) and Garlic Factors (Natural Factors). Garlic has been shown to be an effective germ killer. It helps to preserve meat, keeping it fresh 2 to 4 times longer than meat that is not treated with garlic.

While it was used to keep away vampires, garlic has been shown to kill parasites in the body. With so many uses, it should be on the menu of every household. Here's a quick list of its benefits:

- It acts as an antiseptic

- Fights infection

- Contains chemicals that prevent cancer

- Thins the blood and reduces the chance of clotting in high-risk heart patients. This is especially important for diabetics.

- Lowers blood pressure

- Reduces LDL, the bad cholesterol

- Controls triglycerides

- Stimulates the immune system

- Acts as a decongestant

Tuberculosis is one of the diseases that is mounting a comeback and garlic is particularly effective in preventing it It is effective against botulism, diarrhea, dysentery, pneumonia, staph and typhoid and is a more effective germ killer than penicillin or tetracycline.

Vinegar: Real vinegar is raw and unpasteurized. It's rich in organic acids, friendly bacteria, pectin and acetic acid, which helps to slow down the emptying of the stomach. This translates to less of a rise in glucose levels. It is rich in 22 of the essential minerals for human health and apple cider vinegar contains 19 of these minerals in the right amounts. Potassium is one of those essential minerals. Just 2 tablespoons of vinegar can slow the emptying rate of the stomach as much as 30% and drop the sugar spikes that occur after eating by about 30%. For good health, take 2 teaspoons of apple cider vinegar twice daily before a meal, every morning, or before going to bed. Mix vinegar in a glass of warm water and stir in some raw honey and a drop of lemon juice to make it more palatable. It has been shown that those who took vinegar before a meal had a 25% reduction in blood sugar levels than those who took no vinegar before a meal. Those who took vinegar also experienced weight loss after just 4 weeks. On average, they lost 2 pounds while a non-vinegar group lost nothing.

The store bought vinegar is often more acidic and you'll discover that the raw, unpasteurized version is more palatable.

Onions: Closely related to garlic, onions, cooked or raw it helps to lower blood sugar through an active substance called allyl propyl disulfide which is also found in garlic. This substance helps to prevent the liver from deactivating insulin so it stays longer in the bloodstream where it can lower blood glucose.

The higher the dose, whether taken in a raw onion or powder form produces the greatest effect on blood sugar. Onions are effective both raw and boiled. Like garlic it helps to reduce cholesterol and blood pressure. Diabetics should take liberal amounts of both onion and garlic.

Colorful Vegetables: As we age free radicals (pro-oxidants) increase in the body stealing electrons from the tissues of your heart, blood vessels, brain, cell membranes and your DNA. This process is particularly pronounced in diabetics and leads to premature aging. You can slow down the process by consuming more foods high in antioxidants. Most antioxidants are found in colored vegetables and fruits.

The deeper the greens and reds, the better the anti-oxidant value; plants have to stay in the sun all day and need some protection against free radical damage. Their protection lies in the form of their color. Bioflavonoids and carotenoids protect plants from free radical damage. There are over 20,000 bioflavonoids and over 800 different carotenoids. Deep green vegetables like spinach and collards provide more protection than does iceberg lettuce, which is light in color. Berries, such as raspberries, red grapes, boysenberries, red peppers, carrots all contain a great deal of antioxidant value that can help you in your fight against free radical damage. The more dark red the tomato is, the better it is for you.

Brewer's Yeast: Both glucose tolerance facto and insulin is required to move excess glucose into the cells. GTF is often lacking in diabetics. Niacin and chromium are two important elements to help sensitize the cells, but both are missing in the diabetic diet. The richest source of GTF is found in brewer's yeast, the same stuff used to make beer. The taste is bitter and not very appealing, but it can be mixed with a blended shake of orange juice, powdered protein, flax oil and lecithin or sprinkled on breakfast cereal.

Diabetes Diet

Cinnamon: Cinnamon, cloves, turmeric and bay leaves have a measurable impact on making insulin more effective. Cinnamon is clearly the best and also contains no calories. While the cinnamon in your spice cabinet helps a little, its effect quickly becomes inactive by the saliva in your mouth. The best way is to take the liquid form of cinnamon as you find in your local health food store. Or buy cinnamon sticks and boil one in the water you use to make your tea or coffee. ½ a teaspoon of cinnamon a day can make cells more sensitive to insulin. Research has shown that after 40 days of taking various amounts of cinnamon extract, diabetics experienced lower blood sugar spikes after eating and major improvements in heart health. Glucose, triglycerides and LDL cholesterol levels all decreased.

Grapefruit: While grapefruit interacts with several prescription drugs, the fiber in grapefruit helps against cholesterol buildup in the arteries. Grapefruit juice, on the other hand, lacks fiber. Take a real grapefruit, quarter it, peel, and seed and eat. If you're looking for a sweetener, use raw honey or natural sweeteners such as stevia and Xylitol. Red grapefruit is rich in carotenoids and bioflavonoids. The fruit helps against the sharp rise in blood sugar that often occurs after a meal.

Soluble Fiber Foods: Our ancestors consumed a diet of 50 to 100 grams of fiber every day of both soluble and insoluble fiber. Our diet today consists of less than 20 grams, most of which is insoluble. Soluble fiber is important in that it forms into a gelatinous mass in the intestines, which slows down the absorption of glucose into the bloodstream and improves the course of type 2 diabetes. To get more soluble fiber, simply eat more vegetables such as okra, Brussels sprouts, peas, broccoli, carrots, oats, and beans.

Spinach, kale and collards are good sources of lutein, a carotenoid found in large quantity in the lenses of the eyes. Consuming these foods can help against the onset of blindness that affects a great number of diabetics.

Green Foods

Green foods refer to green tea, and products that contain dehydrated barley grass, wheat grass or algae sources such as Chlorella and spirulina. You get the benefit by mixing with water or juice. They are packed with phytochemicals, especially carotenes and chlorophyll. While you can grow your own, it's easier just to get them at your health food store. Some of the best products are: Greens Plus; Enriching Greens and ProGreens. Drink one or two servings per day 20 minutes before or 2 hours after a meal. Green tea, orange and cranberry juice contain flavonoids, which help fight inflammation. Drink more green tea than coffee.

Dietary Fiber

Fiber supplements have been shown to enhance blood sugar control. This is no surprise when you consider that the diet of most Americans is low on fiber and high in saturated fat and sugar. The best fiber sources for reducing after meal blood sugar levels, lowering cholesterol and promoting weight loss are those that are rich in water soluble fiber, such as Glucomannan, psyllium, guar gum, seaweed fibers and pectin that promotes weight loss. If you take fiber supplements be sure to drink plenty of water. Take 1 to 2 grams of soluble fiber before bedtime and slowly increase the dosage to 5 grams to reach a full dosage of 20 grams. 24 to 50 grams of fiber a day can help you improve blood sugar levels. It has been shown that a high fiber diet is as effective as some diabetes medications.

Diabetes Diet

Legumes such as chickpeas, cannellini beans, kidney beans and lentils are a great source of fiber. You can replace beef as an alternate source of fiber. Low fat, low calorie and high proteins help to reduce the risk of diabetes and heart disease.

PGX: It stands for PolyGlycoPlex and is a collection of highly viscous soluble polysaccharides that acts to develop a higher level of viscosity and expansion in the stomach than regular sources of fiber. PGX lowers postprandial blood glucose by 20% and lowers insulin secretions by 40% A typical dose of PGX should be 1000 mg three times a day with meals.

Touchi Extract: It's a fermented soybean product that's been in use in China and Japan for over 3000 years. It possesses high levels of naturally occurring alpha-glucosidase inhibitors.

Mulberry Extract: Highly regarded in Chinese and Japanese medicine, it possesses significant hypoglycemic effects in animal studies. It has been shown to reduce the amount of damage to cell membranes of red blood cells, a significant antioxidant effect.

ABOUT THE AUTHOR

As I am a diabetic myself, I have read extensively on the subject, looking for natural ways to control my diabetes. There is a lot of information that is misleading, most of which is backed by and promoted by big pharmaceutical companies whose interest is only to sell drugs regardless of what they may do to your health. The fact is that there is no such thing as a safe drug and never will be.

Your body and mind were never meant to take in chemicals foreign to it. Pumping your lungs with cigarette smoke, breathing in toxic car exhausts and industrial pollution adds more enemies than your immune system can handle. With a lifestyle of fast and convenient food we are fast losing the battle for health.

More people as they get older are experiencing more diseases than ever before. It's sad to see our nursing homes filled with debilitated patients whose only hope is to die. Old age should be vibrant and there are those who live to a ripe old age with all their reasoning faculties intact. Study them and you'll find that an active lifestyle and natural food are what keeps them healthy. Old age does not mean senility and loss of function!